Energize
Your Brain...

Change Your Life.

An Introduction to
Exercise With Oxygen Therapy

Jeffrey Donatello, DC

Foreword by Michael Johnson, DC, DACNB

To my Mom & Dad,
whom I am forever grateful.
By raising me the way you did,
you laid a foundation within me
for a lifetime of exploration, adventure
and most importantly happiness.

Contents

Intended Use Statement: The content of this book is for informational purposes only. It is not meant to treat, diagnose, prevent or cure any disease. The purpose of this book is to explain how Exercising With Oxygen Therapy can benefit you, not specifically treat illness. It is the responsibility of the reader to comply with all state and federal laws when utilizing an oxygen concentrator. And most importantly, this therapy should be used only under the supervision of a competent therapist or doctor.

Foreword

I have been using oxygen and exercise with oxygen therapy in my clinic for over the past 13 years and it has greatly enhanced the care that I provide to my patient population. Quite simply, using oxygen therapy in my practice allows my patients to heal faster.

Over the past 3 years, I have been teaching the use of oxygen therapy to over 1,000 chiropractors worldwide.

Energize Your Brain . . . Change Your Life is one of the best books that I have found on the use and benefits of utilizing the healing powers of oxygen. Dr. Jeff Donatello has taken complex information and condensed it into a very easy-to-read, fast-paced format.

It is my hope you take Dr. Donatello's words in his book to heart and start a program of exercise with oxygen therapy very soon.

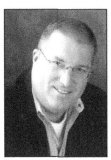

Dr. Michael L. Johnson
Board Certified Chiropractic Neurologist
Author of *What to Do When the Medications Don't Work?*
A Non-Drug Treatment of Dizziness, Migraine Headaches,
Fibroymyalgia and other Chronic Conditions.

Introduction

Why Exercise With Oxygen?

There are many ways to exercise. Turn on the television late at night and every other channel has an over-the-hill movie star promoting the newest gadget or machine promising you ripped abs or instant weight loss. While anything that gets your heart pumping is probably a good thing, the type of exercise you are going to learn about in this book is different from everything else you have ever experienced. And it's all because of one word. Oxygen.

I think Dr. Majid Ali, renowned pioneer in the study of oxygen put it best in his book, *Oxygen and Aging*. In it he simply states, "oxygen ushers in life." Of all the healing substances found on our planet, without oxygen, human beings do not exist.

Oxygen is everything to us; it's the pilot of our immune system, a robust blood cleanser, the strongest anti-oxidant and a vital hormone. It's so important, we can't live long without it. Humans can survive without food for weeks and we can get by (barely) without water for days, but if we lose our oxygen supply, we meet our maker in five to ten minutes.

As we age, our brain cells slowly become less efficient at utilizing oxygen and the cells become more and more dysfunctional. This is a process we all must go through. But what if there was a way to slow this process down? What if there really is a fountain of youth?

There is one fundamental law in life. Everything either grows or it dies, and the human brain is no different.

Take 95-year-old Kansas native Nola Oches. In 2007 she became the world's oldest college graduate to walk across the stage at Fort Hayes University to receive her masters degree in history. The following week, she was interviewed by Jay Leno on the *Tonight Show* and asked what she was going to do with her degree. Her face aglow, she told Jay "she wanted to be a storyteller on a cruise ship." At 95.

Nola is a perfect example of how jogging your gray matter with mental exercise will help your brain continue to grow at any age. The term for this is neuroplasticity. Our brains are like our muscles. If they are properly activated and fueled, they become more efficient.

On the other hand, if we do nothing to keep our brains active, as we get older, the ability to oxygenate our body greatly diminishes, leading to our demise.

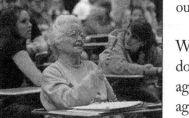

Nola Oches

What if we could at least slow down this primary cause of aging? I am here to tell you aging can be reversed up to a point, using a breakthrough technique called **Exercise With Oxygen Therapy** (EWOT). In the upcoming pages of this book, I will explain how, if properly implemented, exercising with oxygen can lead to life-changing results.

As you read on, keep in mind that exercising with oxygen is a safe and effective therapy based on proven physiological principles. Some may see results very quickly, feeling euphoric after their first treatment, while with others, it takes more time.

I always like to tell impatient patients, "If you plant a tomato seed in a garden, you don't see tomatoes the next day." You need to water and nurture the seed in order to reap the benefits.

Dedicate time and energy toward exercising with oxygen and you have the potential to do great things to your body.

PART ONE

In the Beginning

In the Beginning

"Deep breathing techniques which increase oxygen to the cells are the most important factors in living a disease-free and energetic life. Remember, where cells get enough oxygen, cancer will not, cannot occur."

—Dr. Otto Warburg, President, Institute of Cell Physiology
Nobel Prize Winner

There are all sorts of theories as to the evolution of man. The subject is debated heavily, but one thing scientists do agree upon is that as humans developed, we moved around a lot. The rainforests we started out in as a species incubated us well. They were warm and humid environments full of food. But then the climate started changing and our food sources dried up forcing our ancestors to adapt or die.

Out of the relatively safe jungle they ventured onto the arid plains of Africa. Here our predecessors had to roam around in order to find food. In doing so, their brains needed to learn quickly or they would be eaten by lions and leopards.

The average person 40 thousand years ago would walk 10 to 12 miles per day. This meant our brains developed in an oxygen rich, visually stimulating environment.

Fast forward to our modern society and ask yourself just how crazy it is that we now try and teach our kids in cramped classrooms with poor ventilation and no windows. Or just as bad, that we try to be productive in jobs that squeeze us into little window-less cubicles.

If our brain is to grow and heal we need to get oxygen to it and that is why Exercising With Oxygen Therapy is so important.

DEPRESSION CURED

My first patient to exercise with oxygen in our office was a 52-year-old man named Roger. Once or twice a year his back "goes out" on him with horrible consequences. He says it feels as if someone is sticking a knife in his back. I was told that EWOT could quicken the healing process and asked him if he would like to try it. At this point, Roger would have smothered hot mustard all over his body if it were to ease his pain. So we started him on the therapy.

If you opened up the dictionary to the word diligent, Roger's picture would have been right there. He arrived at the office each morning before our staff at 6:45 a.m., three days a week. He was determined to get out of pain but there was one thing he wasn't telling us. Stress in his life was a real problem and it had been slowly pulling him into a deep and dark depression as recent years passed by. After about three weeks of treatment he seemed to be smiling a bit more even though he was still experiencing leg pain. He no longer had that serious look we were so accustomed to seeing him enter and exit the office with. He was more jovial and fun to be around. Then one day after I closed the door, he asked me, "This oxygen therapy, is it good for depression? Because I really feel good lately." As the weeks went by his leg pain improved and his low back pain all but disappeared but what stayed was his good mood. With his doctor's approval, he started to cut back on his anti-depressant medications ultimately giving them up all together.

I knew we were on the right track with EWOT when Roger's wife came in the office one day. She thanked me profusely, telling me that I gave her husband back to her. She hadn't seen him that happy in years.

How Did My Brain Get This Way?

You may have tried to lead a healthy life up to this point, yet still have areas of your brain that are not functioning like they should be. This may be no fault of your own. Keep in mind, up until fairly recently in modern history, we were too ignorant to realize the need to be kept away from our own human waste. Only after infectious diseases resulted in population-devastating pandemics did we start to put two and two together; if you play where you poop, you get sick.

This is something we now teach to our kids in kindergarten, but as late as the early part of the 20th century, we tossed our feces into the streets via big metal buckets.

Thankfully, we no longer play near our poop, but what about industrial waste and chemicals? The powers that be have yet to make stringent enough laws keeping us apart from these life-sucking substances. Throw in all the toxins we ingest under the guise of "medicine" and it's no big surprise so many of us have sick brains.

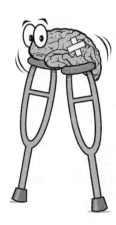

A "sick" area of the brain is an area of the brain full of soft lesions. These are bare areas in your brain where the neurons aren't functioning up to par. The scientific term for this is "transneuronal degeneration" or TND. If you looked at a group of neurons under a microscope that were degenerating, their nuclei might look flabby and be leaking. The entire cell would look withered, in the same way a fruit looks after having been left on the vine too long.

Soft lesions are not easily seen with modern day imaging equipment such as a brain scan or an MRI. This equipment is adept at finding "hard lesions" such as a tumor or a pocket of blood. But if you develop soft lesions, there is hope because as we learned from prior reading, the brain is neuroplastic and can be healed.

The brain slowly develops soft lesions after going through years of stress. The stress can be chemical in nature. For example, living down-river from an industrial plant or sharing a zip code with an unregulated wood-pulp plant may not help you or your longevity.

At the same time, physical stressors can be even more damaging. I have seen many people lead healthy lives then get into a car accident resulting in head trauma. The trauma, while initially minimal, can over years lead to more and more neuron death ultimately leaving a person with a neurological or autoimmune disorder.

And don't discredit emotional stress as it can be just as deadly. A study was done where 68 out of 71 terminally ill cancer patients were found to have lead a life of despair prior to their cancer diagnosis.

CHRONIC FATIGUE ELIMINATED

I had a patient who came to see me two months ago, who complained about constant fatigue during the day, difficulty sleeping at night and a sense of "disconnectedness" as she attempted to navigate through her day. I started her on EWOT three days per week for two weeks. At the end of this time frame, she was ecstatic about her results, describing how she was sleeping through the night, feeling much more energy during the day and more in tune with the world. As a result, she had improved relationships with her family. As an added bonus, she claimed her sex life had improved with her husband for the first time in years.

Dr. Randy Hansbrough
Stuart, Florida

PART TWO

The Origin of Exercising with Oxygen

The Origin of Exercising with Oxygen

Since its discovery by German scientists in the early 1950's, hundreds of thousands of people worldwide have been reaping the benefits of Exercising With Oxygen Therapy (EWOT). But like many cutting-edge techniques in the medical world, our European counterparts are far ahead of us when it comes to this therapy. We are just now here in the United States catching on to the EWOT buzz created in other parts of the world.

Physicist Dr. Manfred von Ardenne is credited with building the atomic bomb for the Russians in the late 1940's. They gave him the Stalin prize and 100,000 Rubles for his effort. Von Ardenne then took the cash prize to his homeland of Germany and built a new institute. There he was able to work diligently on his passion: how the body utilizes oxygen.

How ironic was it that he went from developing a technology with the potential to kill millions of people to one in which he could save millions of people?

Von Ardenne performed blood oxygen measurements on

over 10,000 individuals during his career and figured out a very important fact. In the human body, as stress levels go up, the oxygen content in your arteries goes down.

This is because physical, emotional or chemical stress releases hormones that result in a dramatic lessening of the way your body absorbs oxygen into your blood. And a body that's low in oxygen is a sick body. Did you know that cancer cells can't survive in the presence of an oxygen-rich environment? The cells are anaerobic, meaning that without air, they multiply in abundance. Having this knowledge, wouldn't you think exercising with oxygen should be part of every cancer treatment program? It is in other parts of the world, but not in America.

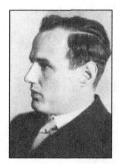

Physicist Dr. Manfred von Ardenne

DIZZINESS GONE

If you work in Maine long enough, it's only a matter of time before you have a lobsterman walk into your office. Captain Glenn was at an impasse in his life when he walked in our door. Every time the lobster boat captain got off his boat over the last month, he would be extremely dizzy. At first, it was only minor bouts of the world spinning around, but after weeks went by, this evolved into him not being able to take more than a few steps off the boat without being so dizzy that he fell down and vomited.

I examined him and determined he had a cerebellum problem. This is the area of the brain that controls coordination and balance. It is also the most oxygen dependant part of the brain and sure enough, the captain tested out to be oxygen deficient. I immediately put him on EWOT. He did not have another attack of dizziness from that point on.

Today, with new technology, blood oxygen is easily measured using a pulse oximeter on the end of your finger. The results are calculated as pO2 or partial pressure of oxygen. For sake of simplicity, let's just say that a healthy individual should see no less than 98% pop up on the oximeter. I have taken thousands of readings in my office and have found that sick individuals or people who smoke tend to have a pO2 of 94% or lower.

Red blood cells carry oxygen to the tissues of the body. Most doctors (including myself) were taught you couldn't pump any more oxygen into the red blood cells as they are already filled to 97% capacity. It didn't matter what you did, very little if any oxygen would be absorbed into them. What Von Ardenne figured out back in the 1950's was that the fluid that the red blood cells float in, called the plasma, could in fact be pumped with oxygen.

Exercising with oxygen results in flooding the plasma with oxygen, not the red blood cells. This increased plasma concentration then pushes the extra oxygen into the cells of the body as the blood flows through it. Even if a little bit of this oxygen gets into the cells of your body, there is a cumulative effect. With the proper amount of EWOT over time, you will increase your pO2 levels, sometimes dramatically.

In order to exercise with oxygen, you need a source of oxygen and this comes from a device called an oxygen concentrator. The invention of the concentrator opened up a whole new potential for the use of oxygen. We now have a safer and less expensive means to obtain it in comparison to utilizing their cousin, the compressed oxygen tank.

An oxygen concentrator is able to take ambient air which is composed of 21% oxygen and concentrate it down to 90-95% oxygen (over 450% more concentrated than the oxygen you breathe).

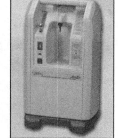

This negates the danger of explosion and the costs of continually refilling a compressed oxygen tank. (To all the nicotine fiends out there, that doesn't

An Oxygen Concentrator

ANXIETY ATTACK HALTED

Stephanie is a 41-year-old woman under extreme stress. She works as a supervisor for a high-tech company. I had been treating her for a right-brain weakness. This kind of brain imbalance causes her to be prone to worry and even anxiety attacks.

One afternoon my front desk buzzed me to tell me that Stephanie called in the middle of a full-blown anxiety attack. Of course she panicked and wanted to come in immediately. When she arrived, her heart rate was 117 (fast). She was breathing shallow and her hands were shaking. She looked like she had seen a ghost.

My treatment was simply to put her on oxygen using my Oxygen Concentrator in a dark room for 10 minutes.

When I came back to check on her, it was literally like a different person was sitting there. She had a smile on her face, her heart rate was down to 79 and she was breathing normally again. The oxygen had stopped the anxiety attack flat in its tracks.

Dr. David Clark
Dallas, Texas
Fellow American College of Functional Neurology
Board Certified Chiropractic Neurologist

mean you can smoke while you exercise.)

A typical concentrator is able to disperse just five liters per minute (5 L/M) of oxygen, which is why two and three concentrators are sometimes hooked together to get the desired flow of ten to fifteen liters per minute (10–15 L/M). This is solely based on your doctor's recommendations.

While exercising with oxygen is very safe, a concern you may hear about is the buildup of carbon dioxide. Medical professionals sometimes have an initial concern here as they are used to treating patients with chronic obstructive pulmonary disorders (COPD) like bronchitis and emphysema. Typical protocol here is to use one to two liters of pure oxygen per minute. The difference between this therapy and EWOT is that COPD patients require oxygen on a continual flow basis. Their lungs do not produce adequate oxygen to a level which supports life and without the extra oxygen they would die. The low flow (1-2 L/M) doesn't build up CO_2 in the way high flow (10-15 L/M) EWOT therapy would if performed continuously, day and night.

This is why exercising with oxygen is done only for short, safe, 20-40 minute, therapeutic amounts of time. That being said, you should never use an oxygen concentrator on your own, unsupervised.

How Will I Feel?

The short answer to this question is you won't know until you try. After the first time you exercise with oxygen, you may feel nothing at all, or you may feel really good. This depends on many factors, one of them being how oxygen deficient you are in the first place. If your partial pressure of oxygen (PO2) was tested to be less than 95%, then the odds are greater that you

"I CAN SEE"

Manny is a retired 88-year-old WWII veteran who was injured on Normandy Beach. He has a myriad of health conditions including heart disease, balance problems, moderate dementia and severe arthritis throughout his body. He has been walking with a walker for four to five years.

He presented to me five months ago after hearing about our exercise with oxygen program. After examination on the first day, he was placed on five liters per minute of oxygen for 30 minutes while exercising with an upper body ergometer. After his treatment he was sitting in the reception room waiting for his transportation service to take him home. All of a sudden he blurts out "Holy cow! I left my glasses at home and I'm able to read this magazine without them. I have been using glasses for 40 years. This stuff really works."

Dr. Lee Barbach
Miami, Florida

will feel more energy quickly. A person who lives with a smoker probably will feel better faster than a marathon runner. But after three or four treatments, the overwhelming number of people say they have more pep to their step, better late-day energy, or that they are sleeping better.

How Long Will It Take?

People starting an EWOT program commonly ask two things.

1. When will I feel better or see results?

2. Are there side effects to the oxygen?

Everyone responds to the therapy at a different rate. From my experience, most people will first notice more energy, some may see it later in the day, and others may notice it in the morning. Many also walk out of our office feeling euphoric having been on the oxygen. This type of feeling makes sense as their brains have just been nourished.

Exercising with oxygen is very safe and there are only minor side effects which occur in just a small percentage of people. The only thing you may notice, especially as you start the program, is that you may develop a slight headache or experience dizziness or nausea. This is rare and happens only to highly sensitive or sick people.

PART THREE

Chiropractors: Leading the Field

Chiropractors: Leading the Field

Presently, chiropractors are the leaders in utilizing EWOT in the United States. As of 2009, over 800 chiropractic offices are utilizing EWOT with their patients. This number is growing daily based on the work of Dr. Michael Johnson, a chiropractic neurologist from Appleton, Wisconsin. He has enhanced a technique called Brain Based Therapy (BBT) and exercising with oxygen is an active part of the therapy. Chiropractors who utilize BBT believe the brain needs two things in order to flourish: fuel and activation.

The brain gets its fuel from two sources. The first from carbohydrates that are quickly converted into glucose. In our carb-laden society, its rare to find someone deficient in carbohydrates, so this is not typically a problem. The second source of fuel is oxygen and as we age, it's more difficult to obtain. This is where EWOT comes in. Keep in mind, however, that exercising with oxygen therapy alone, while beneficial, is only half of the equation. The brain must also be activated or stimulated properly in order to grow and heal.

NO MORE LEG PAIN

Daryl was a successful businessman and former college football player. He was 40-years old but had the fit look of someone much younger. Unfortunately, how he looked and how he felt were two different things. He had a 20-year history of severe low back pain that radiated into both of his legs. They throbbed often and he even had bouts of shooting pain into them. He could not go out to dinner to socialize as sitting for over twenty minutes was excruciating. He was often forced to fly for business and it took him days to recover. He had been to many chiropractors and would get some relief but he had never been on oxygen therapy with exercise before. The very first day he got off the oxygen therapy, his pain went from an 8 to a 0 on a 0–10 scale. It was the first time he had experienced such relief.

Ross Vaughn, D.C.
Vaughn Family Wellness Center

Brain Based Therapists are like CSI investigators. They perform in-depth neurological testing to determine if the cause of your problems are "soft lesions" on the brain. A soft lesion is a group of neurons in a particular part of the brain that are not working up to par. When you look at a soft lesion under a microscope, the cells look wrinkly and old. This happens primarily for two reasons. Either the neurons are not getting stimulated frequently enough or they are not getting the fuel they need. A Brain Based Therapist determines what specific lobe of the brain is dysfunctional, then works at activating it using various therapies.

We have all seen the tests a police officer performs on a suspected drunk driver. He is testing the person's cerebellum to see if alcohol has affected its ability to control the driver's balance and coordination. If someone has soft lesions in this part of their brain, then like a person who has overindulged, they may be dizzy and have poor coordination. The therapy for this would be anything that activates the cerebellum such as vibration, squeezing a stress ball while writing the alphabet in cursive, or specific, one-sided chiropractic adjustments.

The Doctors' Secret

You may be thinking, "If it's so successful, why haven't I heard of it before?" or maybe a better question to ask is "Why doesn't my medical doctor or physical therapist know about EWOT?"

Simply put, it's because oxygen is not a drug.

Pharmaceutical companies make their money from the development of chemical compounds they have created themselves. Conglomerates like Pfizer or Johnson and Johnson can't "own" a natural substance like oxygen, anymore than they can "own" ocean water, so they can't patent it. If they can't patent it, they can't make money off of it. Why spend precious revenue promoting and marketing something that isn't profitable?

This is why you don't see Peyton Manning during a Super Bowl commercial hyping the wonders of oxygen. No one can profit from it so you don't hear about it.

This is the secret not many doctors talk about, but it's the truth. Physicians in our country get much of their continuing education fed to them, literally, during their lunch hours by drug company representatives. Many doctors are overworked and get the majority of their post-graduate education during these lunchtime meetings or weekend seminars, sponsored by the very companies of the drugs they dispense.

And drug reps are all about the bottom line.

They want to influence the doctors in the brief face-to-face time they have with them, to push their product onto the consumer/patient. Do you think for a second the reps are going to talk about a product they don't own? This is why when I talk to local physicians about exercising with oxygen they seem to be in the dark. It's not that they don't want to know about new therapies, it's just not on the agenda. This is why as you start an EWOT program, it's vital for you to discuss it with your doctor. Let them know about the therapy you are choosing to do and keep them apprised of any results you may have. Physicians understand oxygen and its influence on the human body and from what I have seen, are very open to the therapy.

SEIZURE ABATED

Mary was a typical low back pain patient in her late 30's. She worked for the airlines as a ticket agent and came into our office every so often for an adjustment. She was placed on muscle stimulation prior to her adjustment. Five minutes later, my chiropractic assistant ran into my office to tell me that Mary was on the floor. I found her to be on her back with her hands over her head and one of them was trembling. She asked me to move her to a different room so the other patients would not see her having a seizure. I asked her if she did indeed have seizures and she said she felt a Gran mal coming on. I asked her if she took medications and she said only for the severe seizures and she has not had a Gran mal seizure in some time. We immediately put her on EWOT as the seizure had not yet happened but was imminent. Fifteen minutes later, after the therapy, she explained, "I have never had a Gran mal stop without using my meds. Whatever you did worked!"

Michael Ruiz, D.C.
Elk Grove, California

PART FOUR

Is It for Everyone?

Is It for Everyone?

"Oxygen plays a pivotal role in the proper functioning of the immune system. We can look at oxygen deficiency as the single greatest cause of all diseases."

—Stephen Levine, a respected molecular biologist and geneticist, and Dr. Paris M. Kidd, Ph.D., authors of *Antioxidant Adaptation*

In our office we use EWOT on everyone but two groups of people. The first group is pregnant women. Most professionals are not ready to take this risk at this point in the history of the therapy.

The second group some doctors avoid are people with asthma. This is controversial as many doctors give the green light to these patients, but they monitor them closely. Once again, it is up to the individual therapist or doctor to make the decision if they want to utilize the therapy on people with active asthma.

The natural progression of EWOT is to want to be able to do it at home. I do not recommend this, as it is very easy to get too much oxygen. Administering oxygen requires great care. If you don't have enough, you can have severe health problems, but if you get too much you can have worse health problems. For this reason, the use should be monitored by a health care professional.

As the success of EWOT continues to spread, it's inevitable that schemers will attempt to make a quick buck off of it. For this reason, cheap, imitation oxygen concentrators are starting to pop up all over the place in retail markets. These are petite, cute units that while initially attractive due to their small size, only release a purity level of 30-50%. If you use one of these concentrators, you will be disappointed with the results.

The Brain Is a Pig

So why exercise with this therapy? Because the brain is a pig and it needs to be fed. It weighs a mere 2% of the overall weight of the body yet it can demand up to 20% of the total energy usage of the body. When highly stimulated, the brain uses as much oxygen as a fully-engaged quadriceps muscle. If you don't give it what it needs your body will instantly pay the price.

Your brain can't survive on fuel alone. It needs to be activated or stimulated. We all know the saying, "you lose what you don't use." The best way to exercise while on oxygen is to find an action that bombards the brain with the most stimulation. Keep in mind when I mention the "brain" I am actually referring to neurons. They are the stars of the show in the brain. And like any star, they need to be given the proper amount of attention.

RESTLESS LEG SYNDROME

Carolyn is a 64-year-old woman with a five-year history of Restless Leg Syndrome (RLS). She had been placed on several different medications in the last five years for this condition, with little or no success. Carolyn stated her problem would start about 30 minutes after she lay down for the night. For relief, she would have to get up and walk around the house for 10-15 minutes before going back to bed. This went on all night. She started to exercise with oxygen and after her third treatment, she was able to sleep through the night without pain. She is also walking 45 minutes a day now without any pain in her legs.

Dr. Ronald Adams
Statesville Chiropractic Clinic
Statesville, North Carolina

Neurons form the circuits that fire electrical signals, which allow us to think, perceive and react. And when grouped together, the neuron form nerves. Because we rely so heavily on the use of our hands and arms, the brain is intimately connected to the hands via a group of nerves called the cuneo-cerebellar tract.

When you move your arms, these tracts become highly active and rush a load of information to the cerebellum. This information wakes the brain up and forces it to adapt to the new

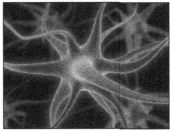

Neuron

stimulation. The brain then connects neural pathways in its attempt to adapt to these new stimuli. This activation "pumps up" your brain and over time, you feel and function better.

We have all seen the sick looking man or woman in a restaurant dragging around a cylinder of oxygen on wheels with a tube running to their nose. These people have a chronic obstructive pulmonary disorder (COPD). Their lungs are scarred and without the extra push of oxygen they would not be able to breathe. The doctors have ordered a prescription of 100% oxygen to keep them going. This flows day and night at 1-3 L/M.

When you exercise with oxygen, you use 3-10 L/M from an oxygen concentrator, which generates 90% oxygen, not 100% oxygen. Some doctors will even raise this level up to 15 L/M. The major difference is that it is performed in short sessions anywhere from five to forty-five minutes in duration. In this way neurons in the brain are nourished yet the body doesn't have time to elevate the carbon dioxide levels to a point where they are dangerous for your body. You see, for every molecule of O2 that goes in, a molecule of CO2 must leave the body. If you drive in oxygen too quickly for too long, the CO2 levels will elevate.

A simple and effective way to use your arms while you exercise is to use an upper body ergometer. You sit down while you do it, and you can easily have access to an oxygen generator on the floor.

Some of the benefits of Oxygen:

Heightens concentration and increases alertness

Enhances memory

Calms the mind

The immune system works harder

Promotes healing and battles aging

The heart gets stronger reducing the risk of heart attacks and strokes

Stabilizes the nervous system

Helps recovery after a hard workout

Increases athletic performance

Encourages better sleep and less daytime fatigue.

It's New Year's resolution time and you find yourself back in the gym hitting the weights. Within two or three weeks you begin to notice those saggy triceps are not quite as loose as they were before. This improvement motivates you to work harder and within two to three months, your clothes start to fit differently and people are commenting on how good you look.

What's going on here?

Your body is simply adapting to an outside stimulus (lifting weights).

You demand more of your muscles and in turn they get bigger and stronger.

FIBROMYALGIA EPISODE

We recently had a woman who suffered horribly from fibromyalgia. She had all the symptoms: leg and arm pain, sensitivity, brain fog, anxiety, depression, vertigo and dizziness. She had been responding to our brain based therapy very well.

One day her daughter called the office just as I was leaving for lunch. The daughter said her mom had collapsed on the floor and she was experiencing every pain she ever had, all at once. She did not want to go to the emergency room, and would I please see her now. I agreed having no idea what I was about to see.

Forty-five minutes later, the patient came into the office looking totally disheveled. She was shaking violently, her hair was stringy from sweating, she was tingling all over and her body was so swollen that there were no spaces between her fingers.

The only thing I could think to do was to put her on oxygen. So we had her stand and receive oxygen from one of our concentrators while she gently swung her arms. This was all she could handle.

It was then that I watched her slowly come back to life. First the color returned to her face, and then the tingling in her body began to subside. After 30 minutes we had her lightly use the upper body ergometer (exercise machine) and put gentle vibration on her feet. 15 minutes later she was back to what she considered normal. It was amazing to watch and obviously a great relief for both of us.

After the incident, the patient, who had fibromyalgia for 26 years, indicated she had these episodes five or six times in her life and each time she went to the hospital. Her specific comment was, "I could have gone to any hospital in the United States with these symptoms and never could have come home feeling like this. I know this because I've already done it and nothing ever worked, not even the medications."

This was the day that as a clinician I realized the true impact of oxygen for the fibromyalgia, chronic pain patient. Oxygen is now a staple in my chronic pain management protocols.

Dr. Martin Rutherfortd
Power Health Rehab and Wellness Center, Reno, Nevada

Our bodies have the potential to change until our last breath, so do our brains. When it gets the proper fuel from oxygen and is activated properly from outside stimuli, it will grow. This incredible ability of the brain allows it to be able to reorganize itself throughout its lifetime by continually forming new neuronal connections. Change your environment, and the brain is right there with you, forming intricate new pathways to help you adapt to whatever you are trying to learn. Do this in an oxygen-rich environment and you learn faster. Humans have been learning this way since we started to walk upright.

PART FIVE

Two Different Ways to "Retire"

"Retire from work, but not from life."

—M.K. Soni

John's Unhappy Brain

I was at a neurology seminar years back and the doctor at the microphone was describing a situation that has always struck me as interesting. He described a man we will call John who worked hard all his life with his hands. John had a tough job on an assembly line but was paid and treated well by the owners of the company. His mind was sharp from the work, but his only real friends in the world were his coworkers.

He stuck with the job for 30 years and as John neared his retirement, he had secret thoughts. The only thing that put a smile on his face anymore was that very soon he would wake up in the morning and do nothing. That's right, after all those years of hard work, he had earned the right to do what he wanted to do. Nothing. So that's what John did. The day after finishing up the leftovers of his retirement cake, he got in his car and drove to the store and purchased a fancy new flat-screen television. He loaded it into his truck and drove down the road to purchase a brand new leather recliner. And this is where he spent his days. Staring at the TV.

He was dead in three years.

Some of you may scoff at this. It was coincidence, you may be thinking. But think for a moment how many people you know who are similar to John. I personally have seen too many to count in my 15 years of practice.

So what killed him?

Doing nothing killed him and this is how it happened.

While on the job, John's mind was constantly activated and challenged. He interacted daily with fellow workers, many of them younger, blue-collar type guys who were quick to bust on the "old" guy. John had to stay on the ball if he was to give it back to them and this kept his mind sharp as a tack.

He also kept his heart rate elevated, while he worked on the assembly line keeping his body fueled with oxygen. In short, he was staying young even as he got older.

Then he retired to 61 inches of wide-screen, high-definition excitement. Having never married, he was alone at home. He lost touch with his coworkers and very quickly the television turned out to be his only social connection. He didn't need to use his hands anymore and he didn't need to move anymore. Worse, he was indoors in a seated position far more often than he had ever been in his life. The amount of oxygen he was taking in paled in comparison to the days he worked. His neurons were screaming for stimulation and he wasn't complying. This slowly led to his death. The moral of the story is, "retire from work, not from life."

So what actually happened? In short, John's brain turned to mush. Remember the fundamental law of life, everything either grows or it dies. As soon as John traded in the brain-

SLEEPING THROUGH THE NIGHT

Lorraine is a 58-year-old home health care assistant who has suffered from severe disc herniation and fibromyalgia for many years. What caused her the most pain was her lack of sleep. I worked on her with many therapies but by far the most successful was using the Upper Body Ergometer (UBE) while exercising with oxygen. Lorraine had the following to say regarding her pain and the success she's had with treatment.

"Basically, I've had fibromyalgia for about 14 years and apart from the muscle problems and everything else that goes with it, one of the worst things is not being able to get to sleep and when I did, to not stay asleep. I would wake up all night long and then never be able to get back to sleep until the early morning hours when I was meant to get up. But since having the EWOT treatments, I have been going to sleep very easily and most of the time I stay asleep all night and it's wonderful. It's really incredible just to be able to sleep.

Dr. Karl Johnson
Shelby Township, Michigan

stimulating environment at his workplace for the brain-numbing environment of his leather recliner, neurons in his brain started to die. This would not have been noticeable at first but over the upcoming months, John suddenly would not be able to remember words quite like he used to. His eyes became vacant, and he was depressed and tired all the time. If he had gone to the doctor, which he never did, he would have been diagnosed or more accurately "labeled" with early onset dementia. Over the upcoming months his health declined even more and cancer set in. He was dead the following year. Would he have gotten cancer while he was working? Perhaps, but knowing cancer loves an oxygen deficient environment really makes you wonder doesn't it? Remember, brain cells need two things to flourish, fuel and activation and John was not getting very much of either of them. So his brain shrank and eventually he died.

It doesn't have to be like this.

MIGRAINE HALTED IN ITS TRACKS

Aleisha is a twenty-four-year-old woman who has had crippling bouts with migraine headaches since the age of thirteen. She was taking powerful medications that she would inject into her arm when the headaches hit. She then would lay in bed for a few days before she could go back to work. Not a great way to live life. All the "headache specialists" had told her she would have to learn how to manage her pain for the rest of her life. On her second visit, she was driven to the office by a friend as she had been in bed for five days with a "killer migraine" that she rated as a 10 on a 0–10 scale. Even the injectible drugs did not help. On arriving, she did not even want to open her eyes. We put her in a dark room and administered three liters of oxygen for 10 minutes. When she finished, she could open her eyes and her pain was now a 6 on a 0–10 scale. We did a few other brain-based therapies and when we were done, her pain was a 2 on a 0–10 scale. She had tears in her eyes when she asked if we could schedule her appointment for later the next day as she planned to go back to work the next day for the first time in a week.

Dr. Robert McCarthy
Greenville, North Carolina

The Eighty-Year-Old Aerobics Instructor

Walk into any senior citizen center and take a look around. There are typically one or two older women who seem to be in charge. These are the ones who are retired teachers or ex-business woman, highly successful and organized in their day, who never lost the zeal for life. They live by the motto, life begins at retirement. While other seniors sit around all day, the ones in charge are like busy bees, motivating the group with endless energy.

This is my friend Peg. She has the same liveliness now at 82 as she did when I first met her at 68. She has an omnipresent smile on her face and is always super excited to tell me about her next project. Whether it's a play or the new lunchtime aerobics class she is organizing, there always is something on her plate.

Another way to put it would be she is always activating her brain. The exact opposite of John, Peg is not letting her neurons die. In fact, by finding new and exciting ways to entertain herself and others, she is actually forcing her brain to be more neuroplastic, continually forming new and complex pathways of growth at age 82.

So, the choice is up to you. Do you take charge of your life and lead aerobics classes or do you sit in front of the television and watch daytime soap operas?

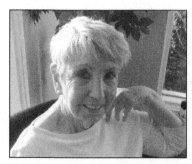

Peg Cadman (aerobics instructor)

PART SIX

The Hidden Answer to Staying Fit

The Hidden Answer to Staying Fit

"Breathing correctly is the key to better fitness, muscle strength, stamina, and athletic endurance."

—Dr. Michael Yessis, Phd., President, Sports Training Institute,
Fitness Writer, *Muscle and Fitness Magazine*

Once you have regained your health, it is time to take your life to the next level and become fit. You are going to be swimming against the tide here in America as the majority of the population is going in the opposite direction.

Over the last 10 years, due to budget constraints, we have started a horrible precedent across our nation. Physical education is being taken out of the curriculum in schools or limited to one day per week.

In short, this is training our kids to be sluggish. And sluggish kids become sluggish adults. You must move in order to thrive and people in America do not move their bodies enough and it shows. As of this writing, close to 70% of the people in the United States are overweight, and one in four are obese. Over 90% of people who lose weight through dieting alone, without exercise, will gain the weight back within one calendar year. That being said, if you don't want to be a statistic and desire to keep the pounds off and get healthy, you must get your body moving. EWOT is a great way to start but at some point you must transition to an at home exercise program. Some of you may want an oxygen concentrator to use at home but, as I mentioned prioir, this is not advisable, as the use of an oxygen concentrator should be monitored by professionals.

Most people start off on fitness programs all excited and raring to go. Unfortunately, their enthusiasm wanes and after a few weeks they fall back into their original habits of being lethargic. This is why every yard sale has a least one piece of infomercial purchased exercise equipment.

I have the hidden answer to this.

Don't exercise, train instead. Last year I was ranked in the top one-percent in my age group in USA Triathlon. This did not happen overnight, nor was I blessed with blazing genetic speed or endurance (my father was an offensive lineman in football). How I did this was years of incremental goal building. Every time I work out, I continually envision myself racing. I have specific goals in mind, which motivate me to get myself out the door each morning to train.

That leads me to another important point. You should train in the morning, not the nighttime. There are two reasons for this.

First, you prime your metabolism for the day when you exercise in the morning. The energy you obtain allows you to focus on the tasks of the day far easier than if you just got up, showered and went to work.

I find that a person who exercises in the late afternoon or at night typically does it based on their schedule. They work out in the evening because they tell themselves they are not a "morning person." Some people may be genetically or hormonally predisposed to not being wide awake early in the morning. For these people, it may be difficult but you can change. All it takes is forcing yourself to go to bed just one hour earlier each day for a month. Within a month, you will find yourself getting up earlier and earlier each morning on your own, and now you have time to exercise. Or should I say train.

Second, by exercising in the evening, you are making other aspects of your life primary and the exercise secondary. When this happens, frequently you won't have time to fit it in at the end of your day as you are too busy. Miss a couple of workouts and the motivation dissipates and you can kiss the exercise routine goodbye.

Don't believe me? Think about all the early morning walkers you see around your neighborhood or on your way to work. Every area has two or three of these morning die hards. Each morning on my way to work I drive by the lady with the Dunkin Donuts coffee cup who walks three miles each way for her shot of Joe. Then there is a "fast walker" with the German Shepard. Every neighborhood has them.

How many of these types of people do you see with an afternoon routine? Watch from now on who is out moving on your way home from work. It will be different people all through the year. This is because most afternoon exercisers drop out.

Setting Goals

Although I am a huge proponent of triathlons, don't go out and sign up for one just yet. First you must purchase a pedometer. This is a small, inexpensive device that attaches to your hip which measures how many feet you have walked over a given time. It's a great way to set personal mini-goals as you walk farther and farther each day. Very soon, you may find yourself parking farther away from the store or climbing stairs instead of using the elevator just so you can see a higher number at the end of the day on your meter. In doing this you are burning calories but more importantly, you are preparing yourself for the next step, signing up for a local 5K run. 5K's have become hugely popular, as every civic group around seems to be organizing one. Each weekend, at least here in the northeast, there is one and sometimes two or three to pick from throughout the year. At just over three miles, everyone has the potential to finish, even if you walk.

Most people's fear about participating in their first 5K is that they will come in last and be embarrassed. They envision groups of fast, fit people snickering at them as they crawl across the finish line, yelling "water, I need water." There is nothing further from the truth. I have directed many of these races myself, and I can tell you the people who bring up the rear get far more cheers when they finish than the skinny, fast guys out in front.

Taking Action

Put down this book for five minutes and go to the website *coolrunning.com*. Find a local 5K that occurs three months from now. Start today by walking 10-20 minutes around the block or close to home without getting your heart rate to a point where you can't finish a sentence without huffing and puffing. Progressively build on this until you can run a few steps. Run/walking is the precursor to actually running. Over the next four to six weeks, strive to get up to 40-minutes per day, four days a week. It's better for beginners to walk/run longer with less intensity, so don't worry about cranking up the speed. It will just cause injuries.

Don't Forget

Make sure you monitor your body, especially if you are over forty years old. You are going to stress it out physically, and injuries will set you back. Find a good chiropractor and a good massage therapist. You are going to need them. All the top athletes get adjusted and have massage work done nowadays. Also, make sure your arches are supported by having good shoes. I use a scanning device in my office to check arch pressure and frequently we find people have lost their arches and need orthotics. Make sure a professional checks your feet, especially if you develop ankle or knee pain early on in your training cycle. Did you notice how I used the words training? You are now an athlete training for a race, not an overweight person trying to trim pounds. Keep this in your mind at all times and very soon, your life will be different.

Epilogue

Hopefully, if you have finished reading this book, you are well on your way to exercising with oxygen and exercising for your good health in general. And you have been fortunate enough to find a practitioner near your home with the proper knowledge and equipment to take you to another level of health.

If you are reading this and you do not have a location where you can exercise with oxygen, then please go to the following resource:

www.lifechangingcare.com

This is a website with well over 800 chiropractors around America who use EWOT in their practices. And above all, please contact me personally if you have any questions concerning the therapy. My email address is *jdonatello@yorkchiropractic.com* and my office phone is 207-438-9339.

Index

Made in the USA
Las Vegas, NV
03 April 2025

20469527R00039